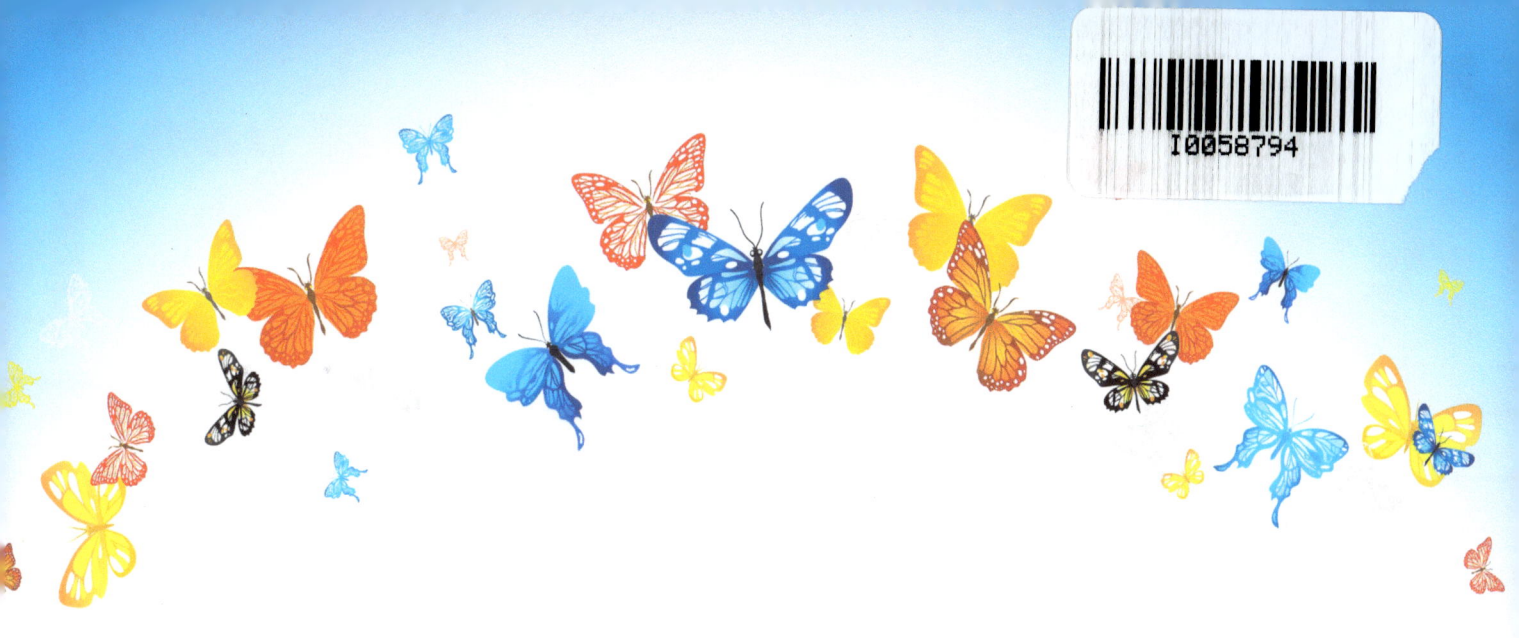

"Amazing Kids' Stories by a Kid"

Part One

By Anoushka Parag Mahajan

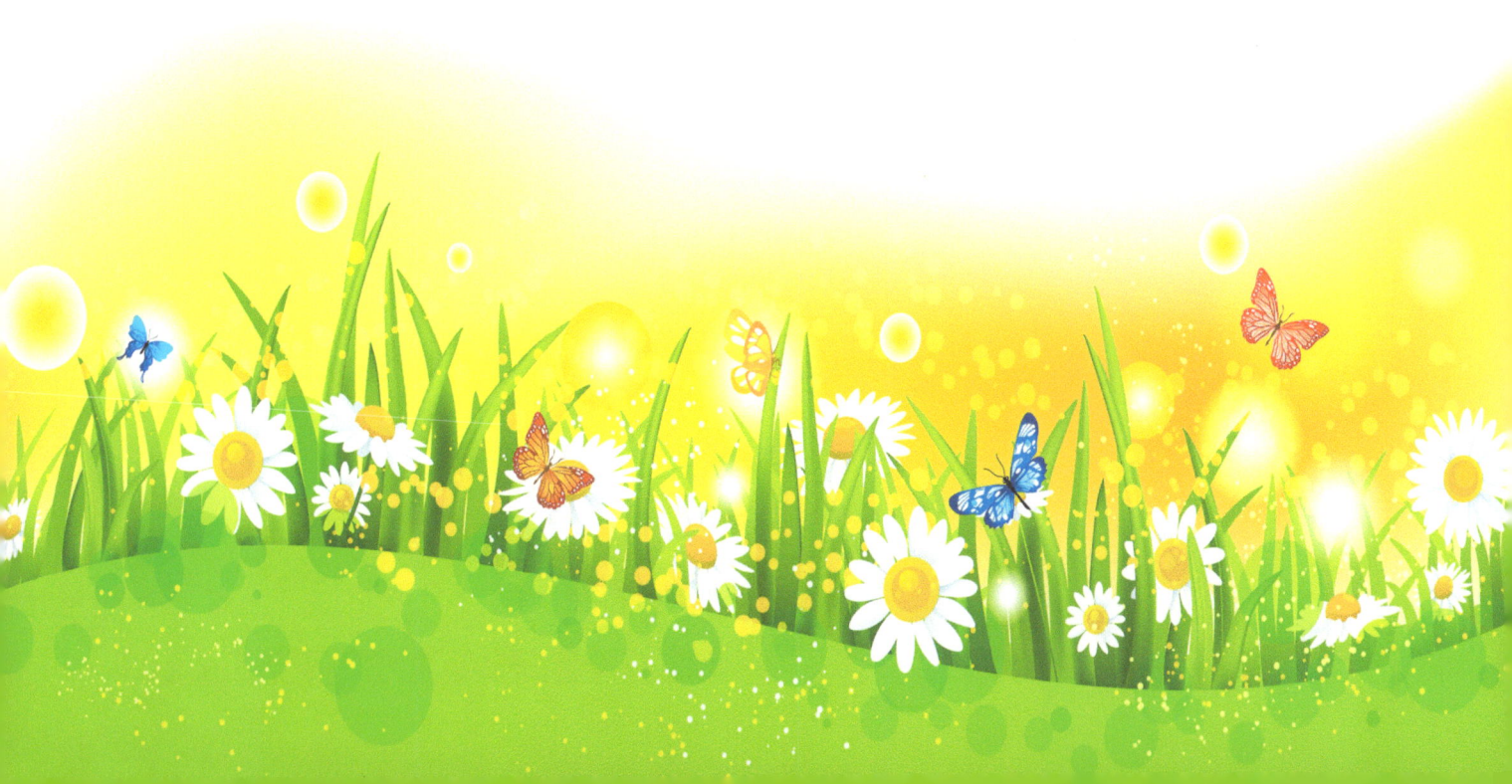

"Amazing Kids' Stories by a Kid - Part 1" Written and Published by Anoushka Parag Mahajan, B3/102, Plot No. 239, RDP-6, Kesar CHS, Charkop Market, Charkop, Mumbai, India - 400067

www.MedMantra.com/apm

Hardcover Print Book ISBN: 978-93-5281-773-3

Paperback Print Book ISBN: 978-93-5281-694-1

E-book ISBN: 978-93-5281-620-0

CONTENTS

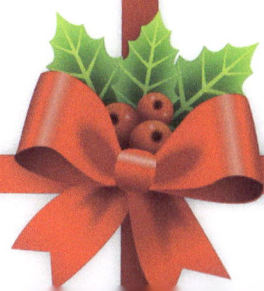

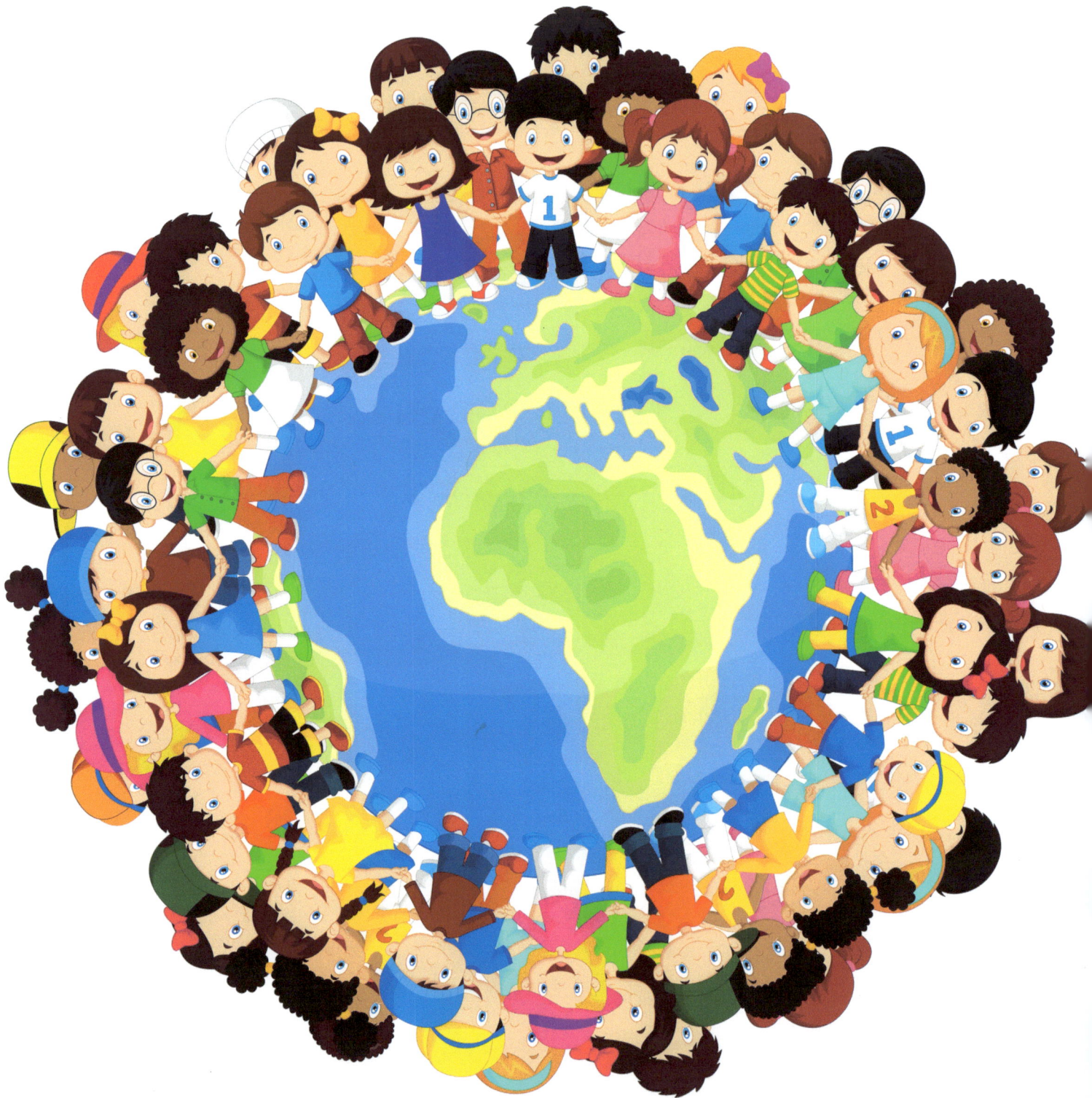

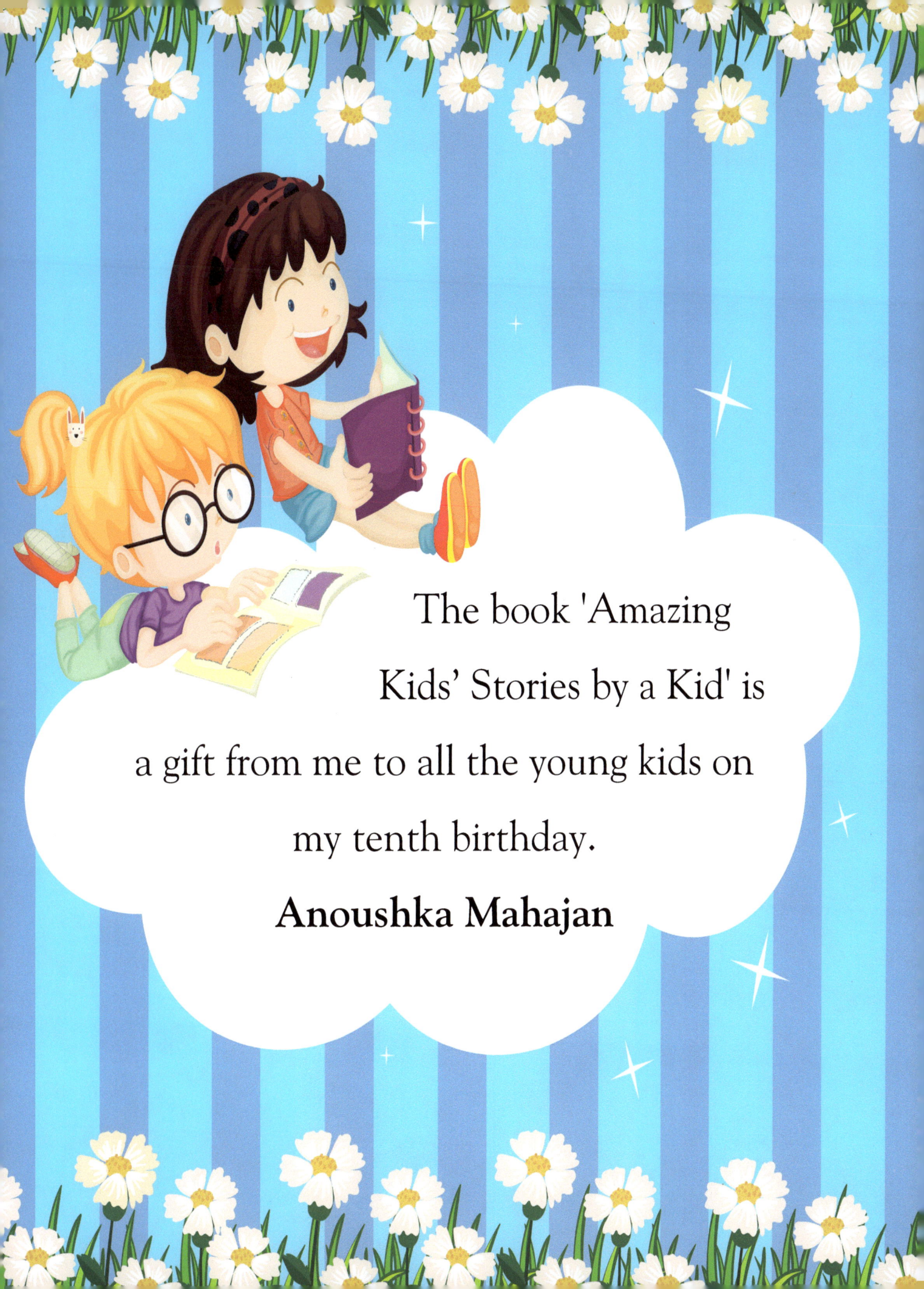

The book 'Amazing Kids' Stories by a Kid' is a gift from me to all the young kids on my tenth birthday.

Anoushka Mahajan

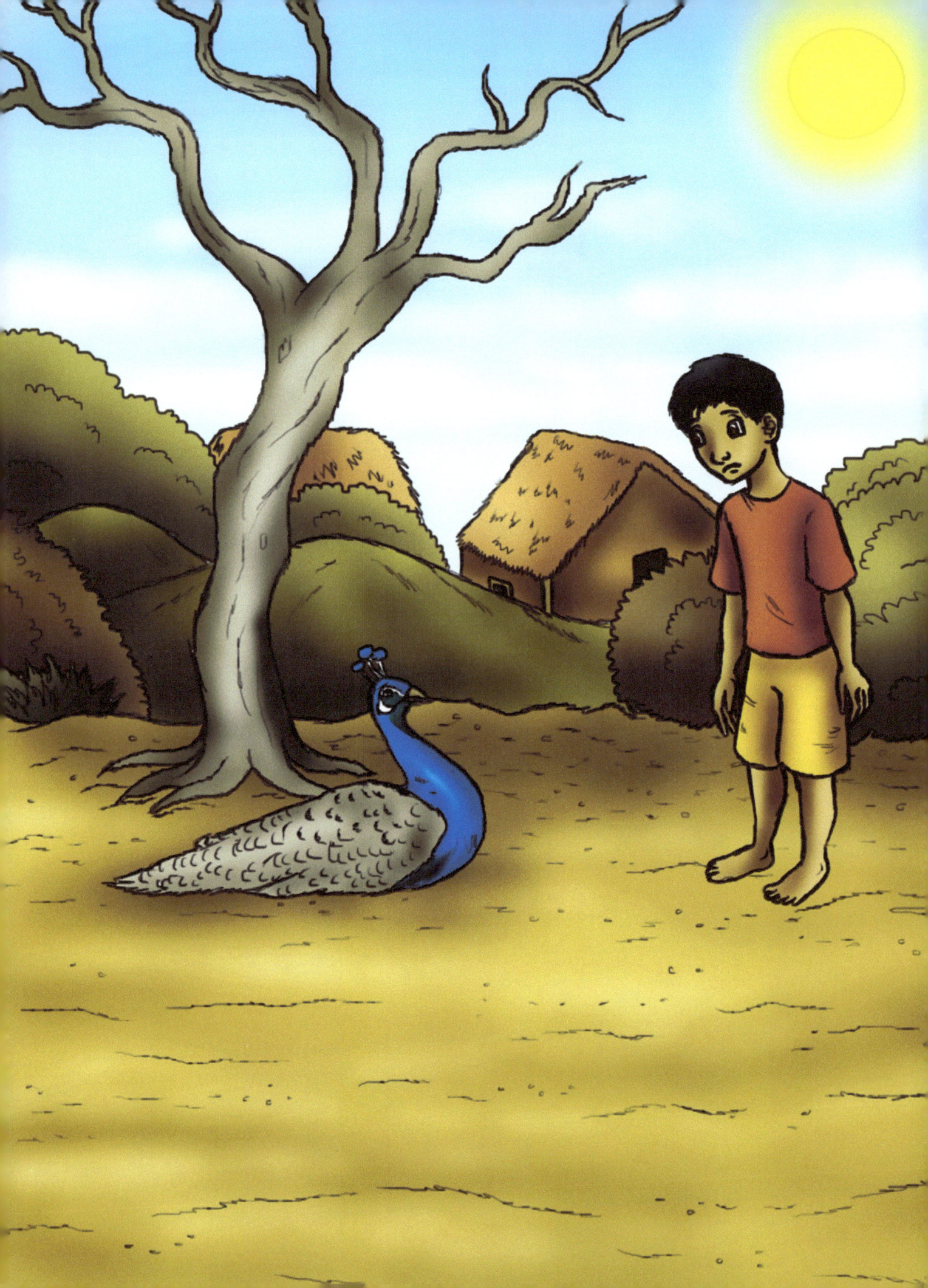

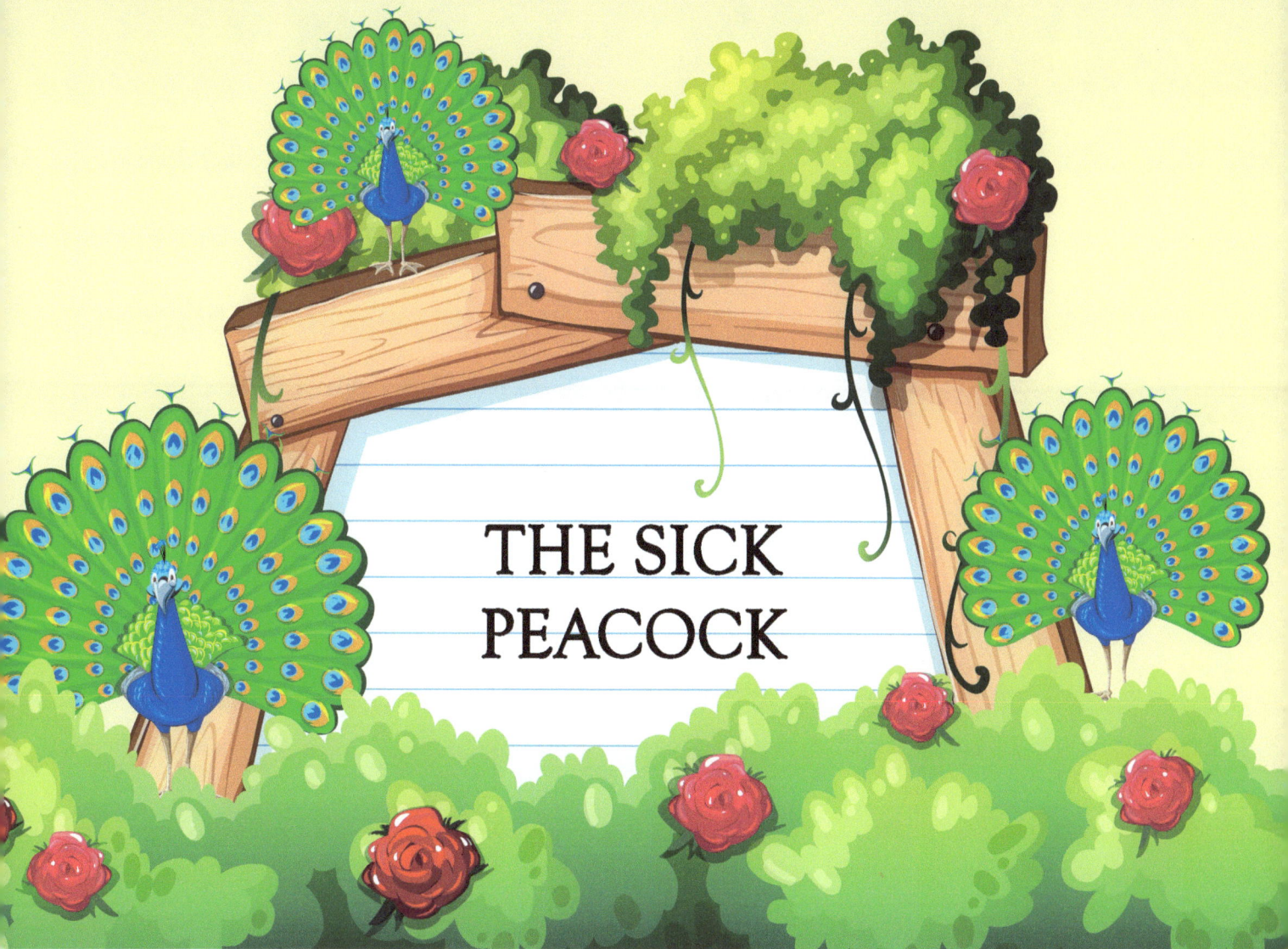

THE SICK PEACOCK

Once upon a time, in a small village by the forest, there lived a very beautiful peacock. The peacock had long, colorful feathers and a pretty blue colored body.

The village in which he lived was rich with plenty of food and water. There was never any shortage of food or water. So, the peacock was always happy, and he danced in the rain. All the villagers admired him.

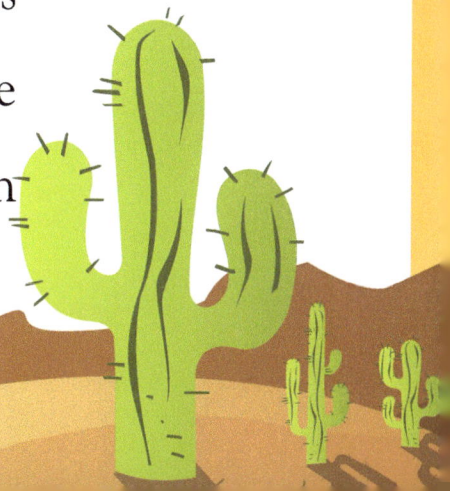

Years passed by, and suddenly it stopped raining in this small village. There was a drought – a long period without rain. As there was no rain, the farmers could not grow crops on their farms. And so, all the people living in this small village and the forest animals and birds did not have enough food and water.

After some time, many humans, animals, and birds died because of the shortage of food and water.

The good people who lived in the nearby village helped them by giving them little water every day. But the water they got from them was not enough, so it was not given to the animals and birds; it was used only by the people.

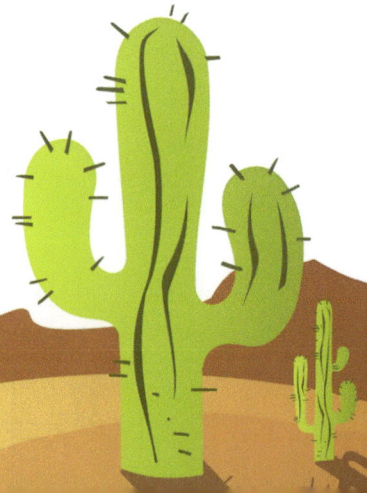

By now, the peacock was very thirsty. Everybody passing by saw the thirsty and sad peacock, and they all were very sad for the peacock. Many people passing by thought of giving some water and food to the peacock, but then they would hold back as there would be less water for them to drink and use, and so they went away.

One day, a little boy saw the sad and thirsty peacock. He ran home and took little water in a small bowl. Not letting anyone see him, he took the bowl with water to the peacock.

But because of the hot burning sun, all the water in the bowl had dried up before the kind boy reached the peacock.

The kind boy went home sadly, as he could not give any water to the peacock.

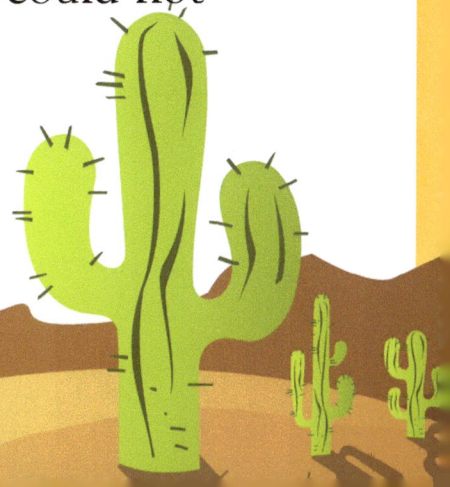

After some years, it rained a lot. All the people were very happy as it had rained in the village after such a long time. All the villagers and the forest animals had plenty of water to drink. Farmers grew their crop, and they had enough food to eat.

But the peacock did not dance in the rain the way he used to, and did not drink water as well. Since all the villagers were so happy that it rained, they did not pay any attention to the peacock.

One day, a kind young man was passing the street, and he was the same man who tried to bring water for the peacock when he was a little boy.

The small boy had studied a lot and had grown up becoming a vet (an animal doctor). He loved animals, and he treated animals with a lot of care and concern.

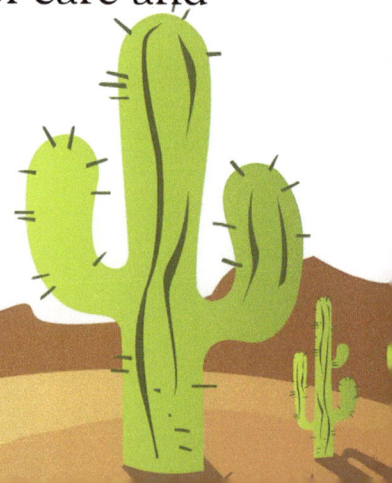

When he saw the sick peacock, he went to him and took him home. He treated the peacock with a lot of care, and looked after him well until it got better.

The young man then recognized that it was the peacock he had taken water to when he was a boy. The young man was very happy that finally, he was able to help the peacock.

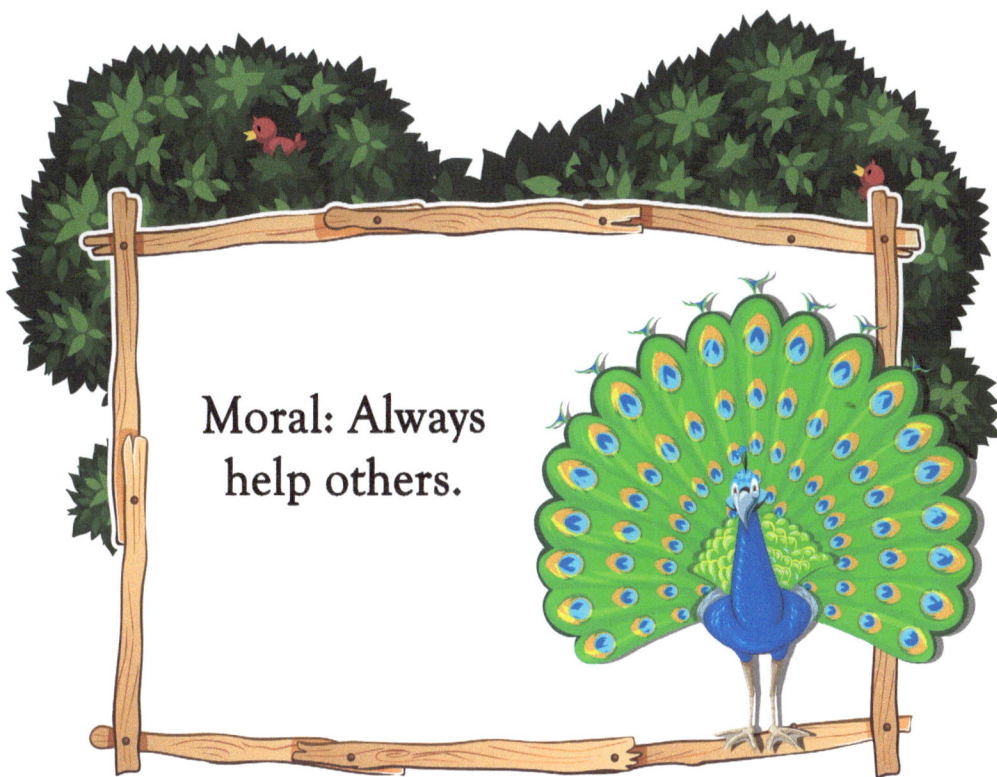

Moral: Always help others.

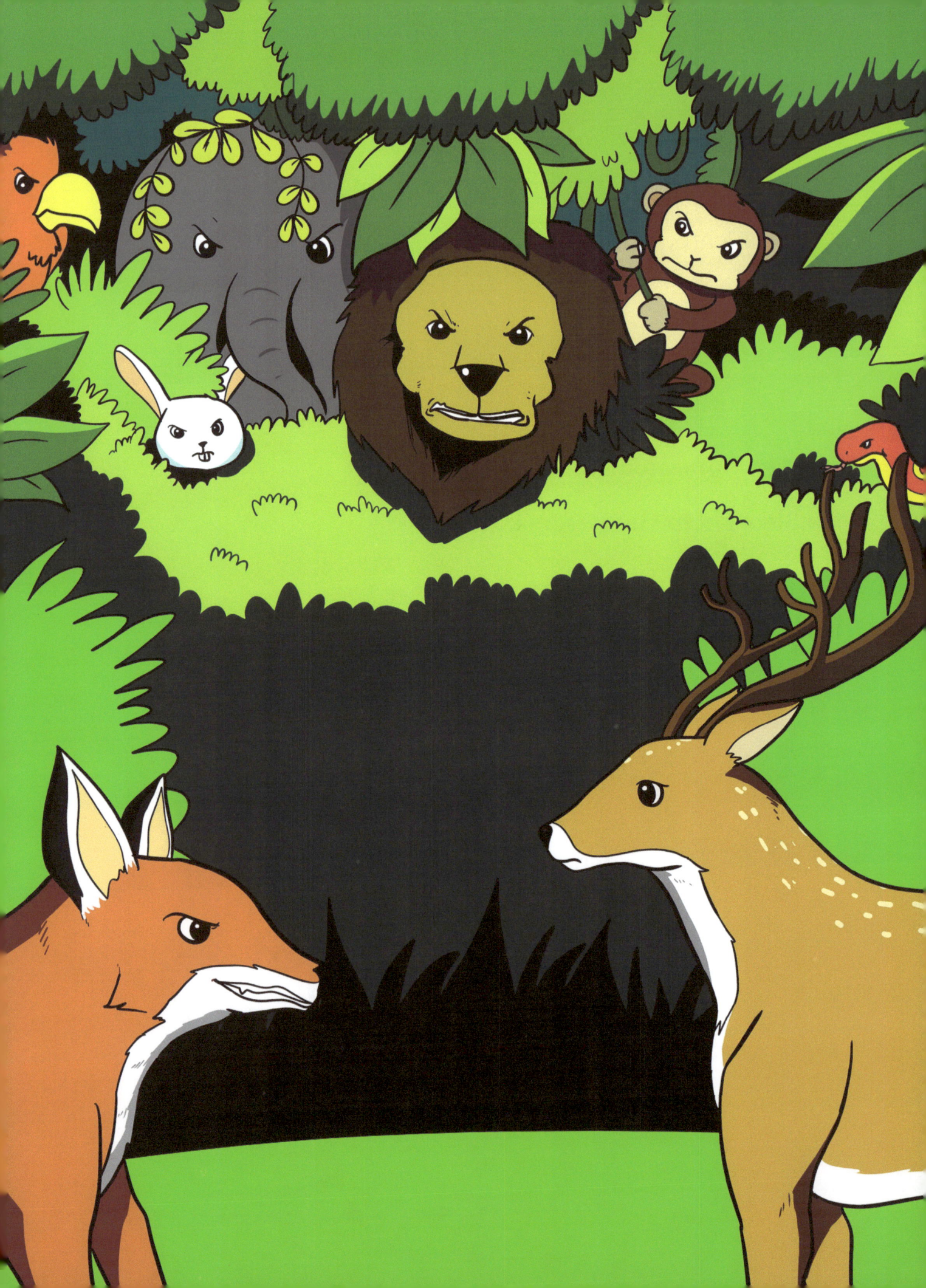

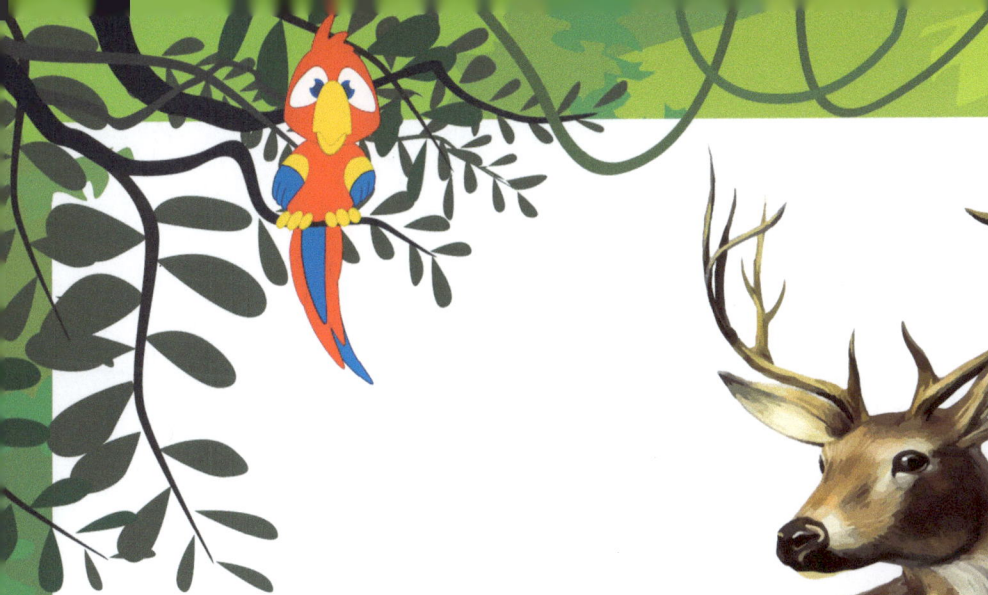

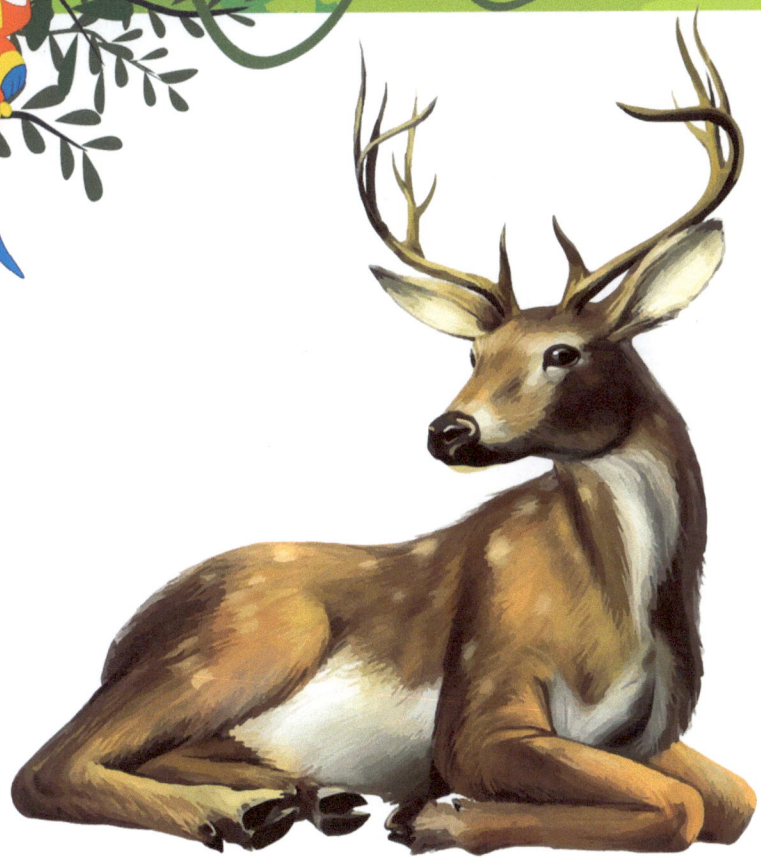

THE KIND DEER

Once upon a time, there was a deer that lived in a large forest. He was a very loving deer. All the animals loved him very much, but only the fox did not like him.

But the fox always behaved very kindly in front of the other animals. So, all the other animals thought that the fox was a very helpful fox. But the fact was – he was not; instead, he was cruel.

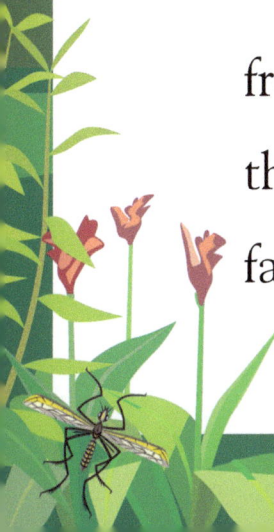

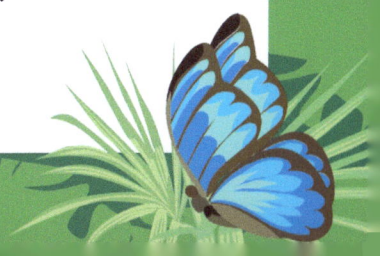

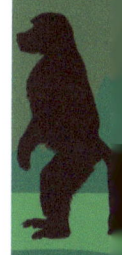

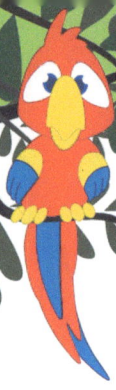

Since the other animals had never seen him behaving badly, they did not know that he was cruel.

Many times, the fox did a lot of bad things to hurt the deer. But as the deer was very kind, he always forgave the fox.

One day, the fox collected stones and kept throwing them at the deer. The fox didn't know that a rabbit was watching his cruel act.

The rabbit hurriedly went and told the other animals about the fox's cruel act. But they did not believe him, because they thought that the fox was very helpful.

On another day, the monkey and the lion saw the fox doing the same thing to the kind deer. Both of them told the other animals what they had seen.

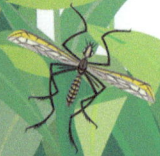

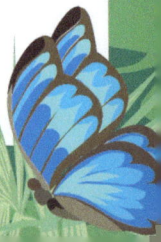

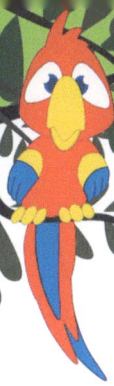

This time the animals began to think, 'Since all of them; the lion, the rabbit, and the monkey are saying that the fox is cruel, there must be some truth in it.'

The other animals said, "Okay, then show us what you saw."

The lion, the monkey, and the rabbit agreed.

The three animals took the other animals to the same place where it happened. All the animals watched for a long time, but they did not see the fox or the deer.

They asked, "Where are the fox and deer? Nothing is happening."

The lion said, "I think since it is late evening, they both have gone home."

The rabbit suggested, "You all come here, to this same place, tomorrow. Come a little earlier than we came today."

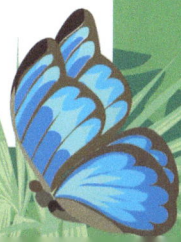

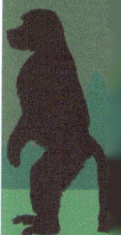

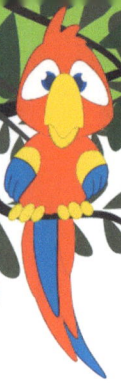

That night, the monkey came again to the same place to see if anything was happening. But when he reached there, he saw that nothing was happening. So, he went home.

However, the lion, the monkey, and the rabbit continued to tell the other animals that the fox was cruel and that they had actually seen him pelting stones at the kind deer.

The next day, all the animals went to the same place, earlier than the previous day, to see whether anything was actually happening or not.

When they reached there, they saw the fox beating the kind deer with stones.

They became very angry with the fox…

They pulled the fox to beat him very badly, but he ran away.

The fox was never seen again.

The kind deer became the king of all the animals.

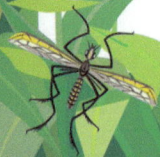

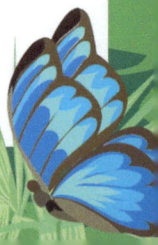

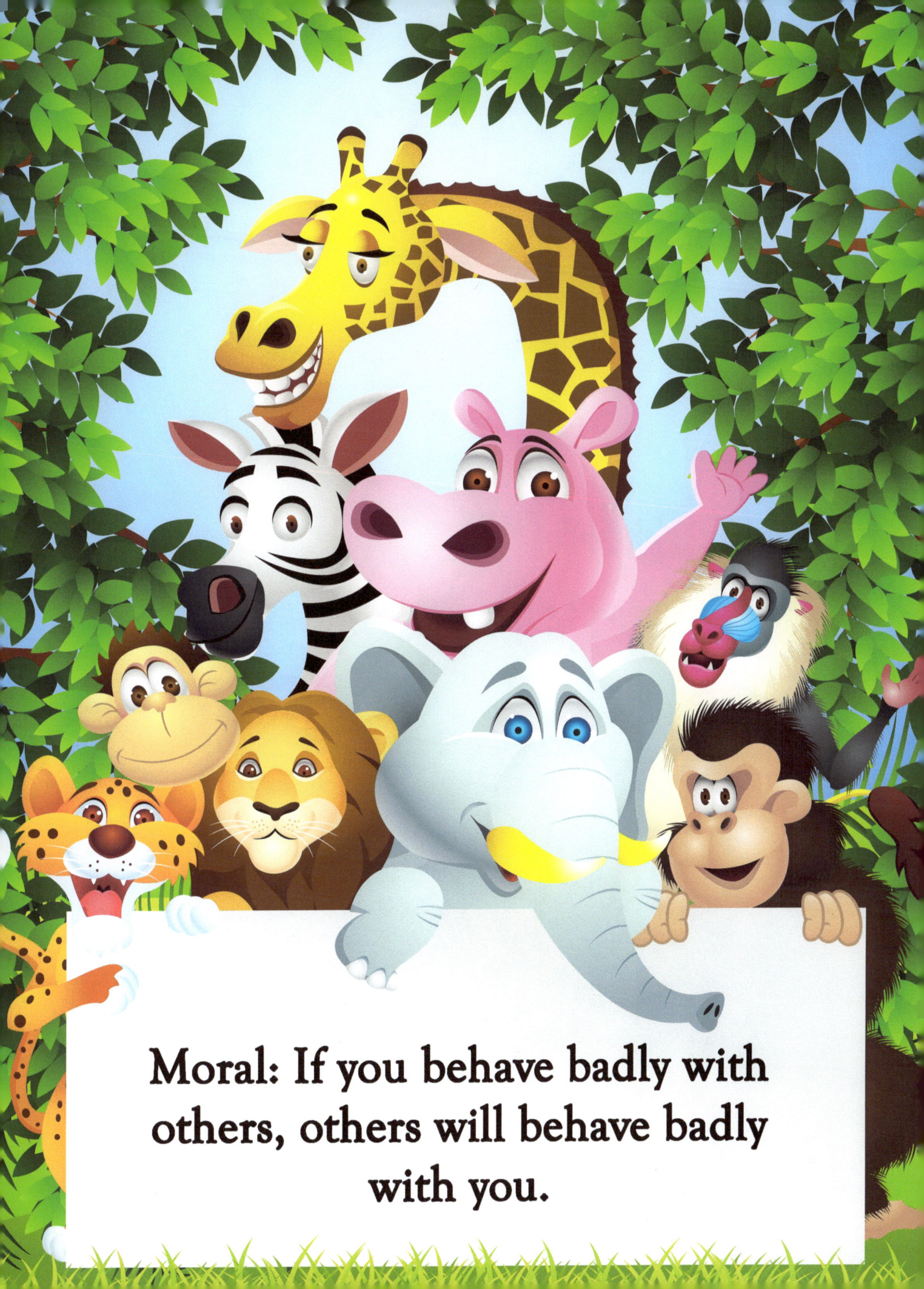

Moral: If you behave badly with others, others will behave badly with you.

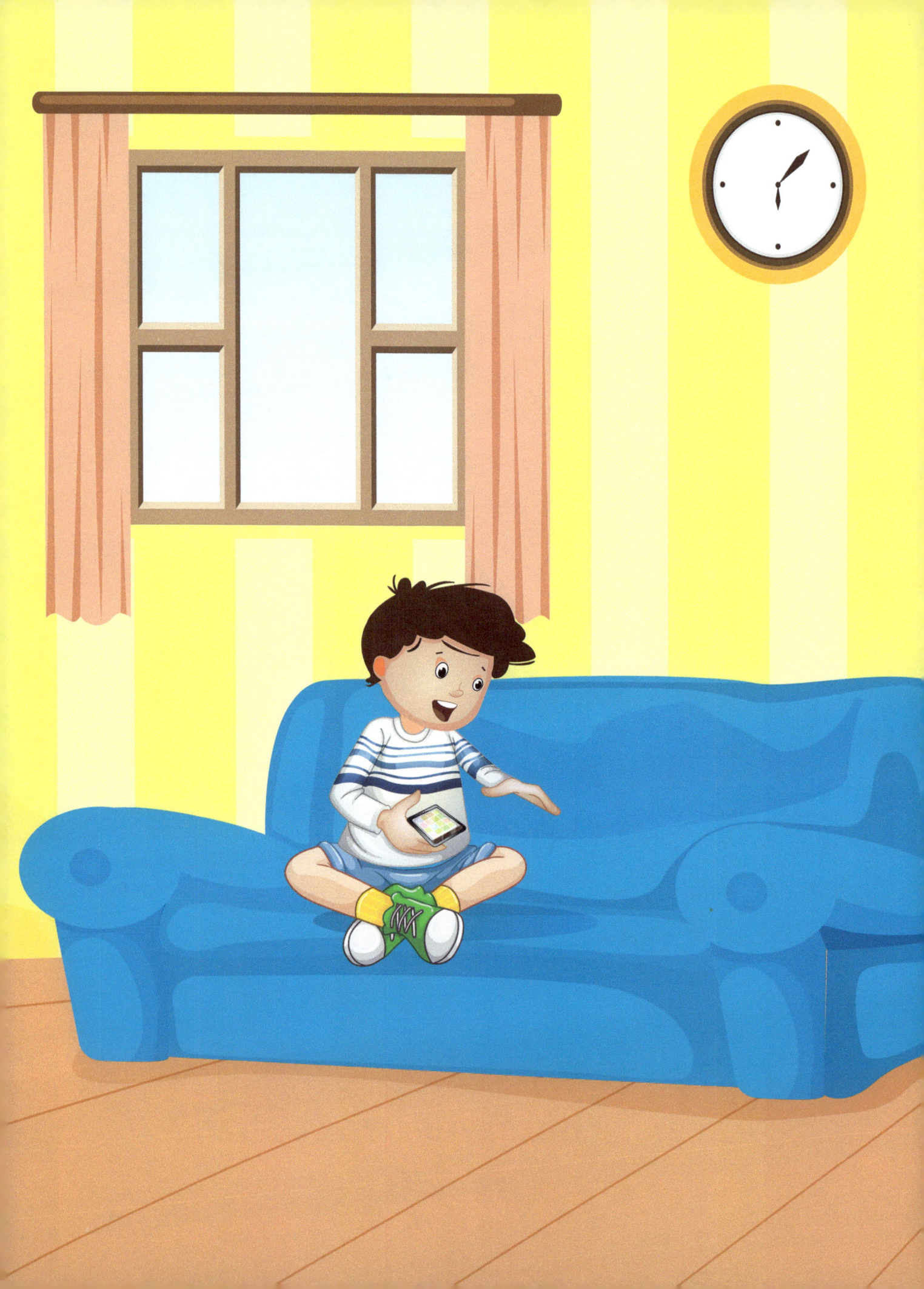

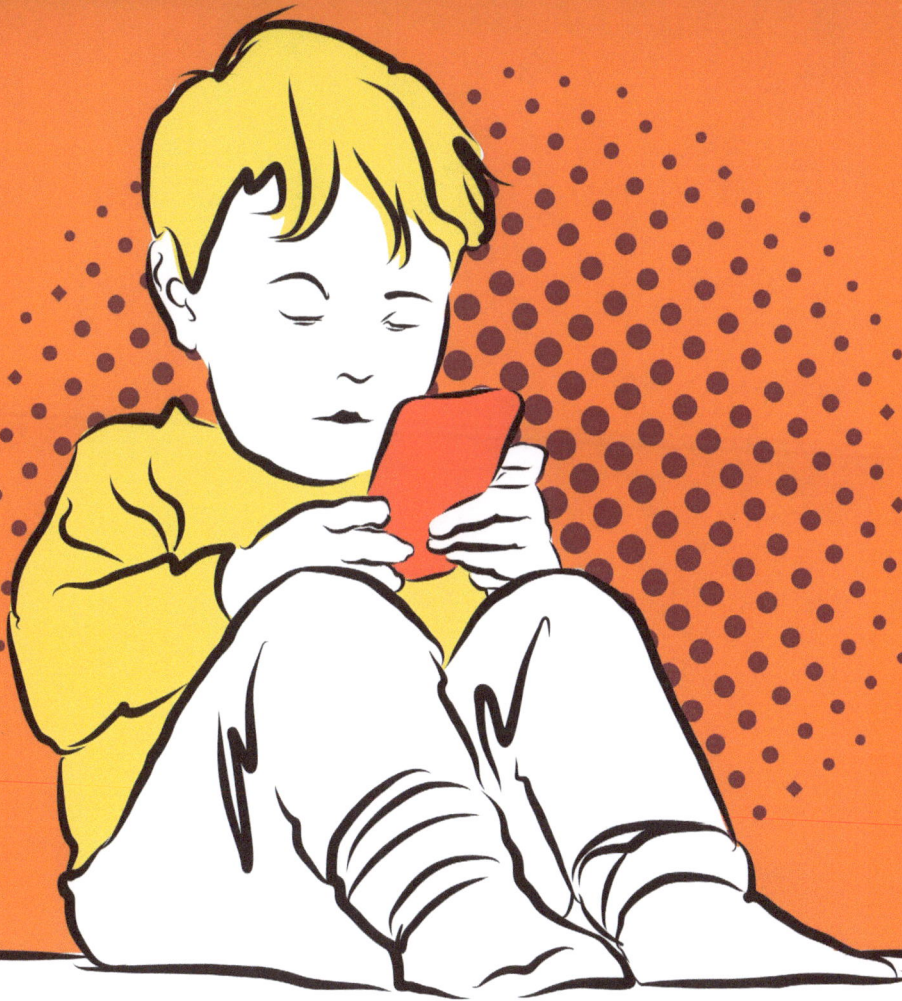

BUMBA AND THE MOBILE PHONE

Once upon a time, there lived a very naughty little boy named Bumba.

It was school vacations, so Bumba was at home.

Bumba often played with his mother's mobile phone. One day, Bumba was playing with his mother's mobile phone, while his mother was getting ready to go to her office for work.

After his mother had left, Bumba continued to play with his mum's phone.

Suddenly, he got an idea...

Being a mischievous boy, his idea was to throw his mother's mobile phone in the dustbin that was outside his home.

Bumba went near the dustbin to throw the phone…

Then he thought, "when my mother throws something in the dustbin, she will see the phone and punish me.'

So, he did not throw the phone in the dustbin.

But, he got another mischievous idea – that was to hide the mobile phone in his wardrobe.

So, he hid the mobile phone in his wardrobe.

Later that day, when his mother returned home, they all had dinner.

After dinner, his mother asked him, "Do you know where my phone is? Or do you have it?"

"No," said Bumba.

His mother said, "Tell me the truth Bumba."

"Mom, I am telling the truth," replied Bumba.

"Okay," said his mother.

Then, it was time for Bumba to sleep. So, he went to sleep.

In the morning, Bumba woke up early. When he opened his wardrobe to wear his clothes, he checked for the mobile.

But it was not there…

He became very frightened. He told his mother, "Mom, when you went for work yesterday, I took your mobile phone and hid it in my wardrobe and, now it is not there."

Bumba started to cry.

His mother told him, "Stop crying 'Bumba', the phone is with me. Yesterday while you slept, I took it from your wardrobe."

Bumba was very surprised to hear this. He asked, "But mom, how did you know that the phone was there?"

His mother replied, "When I was keeping your clothes in your wardrobe, I saw the phone and took it."

Bumba felt very embarrassed about his naughty act.

Bumba went to his room. He sat on his bed and thought, 'I shouldn't have hidden mom's phone in the wardrobe. I should have thought that mom would find it. It was a very silly idea.'

**Moral:
Think
before you
act.**

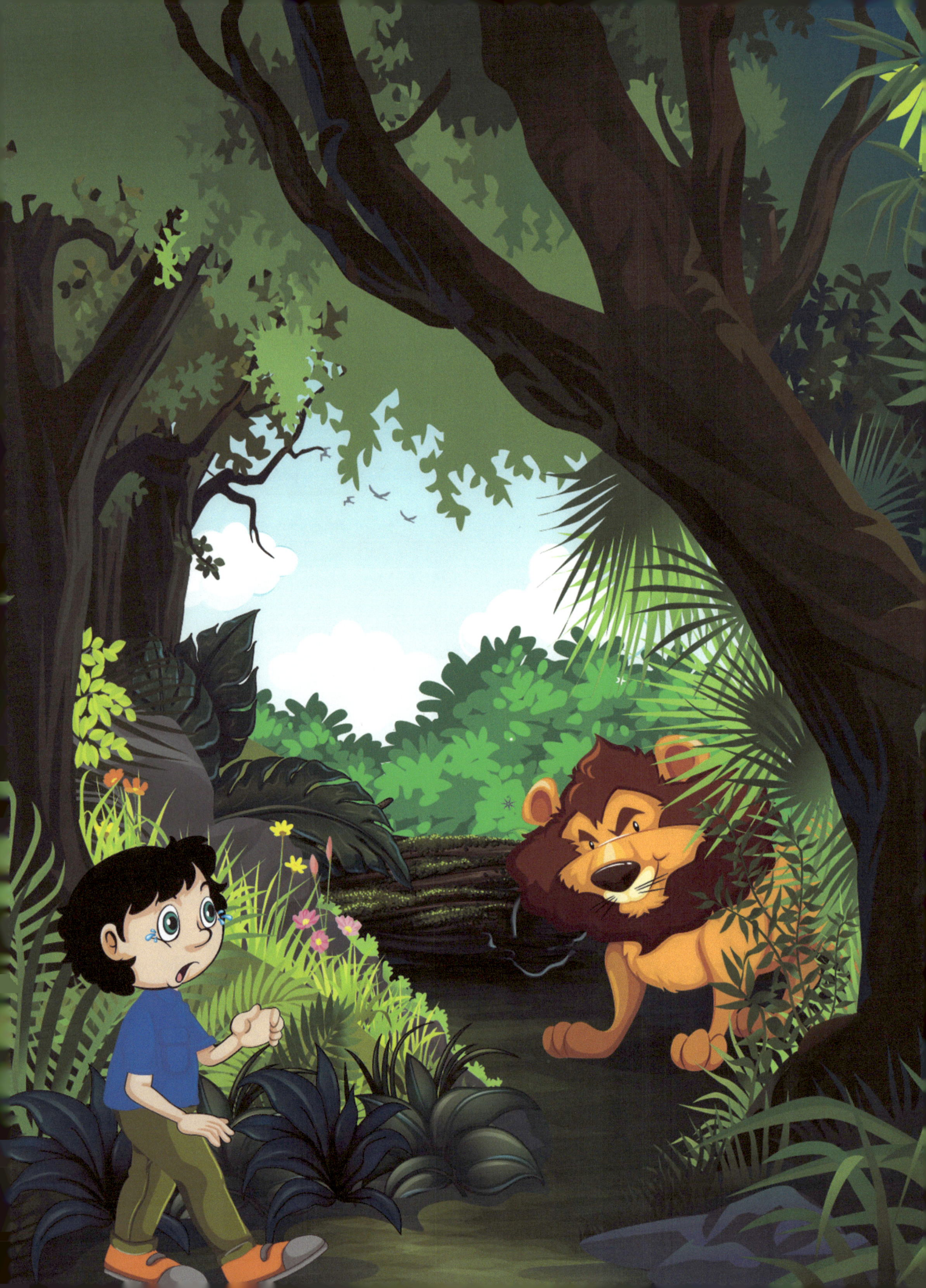

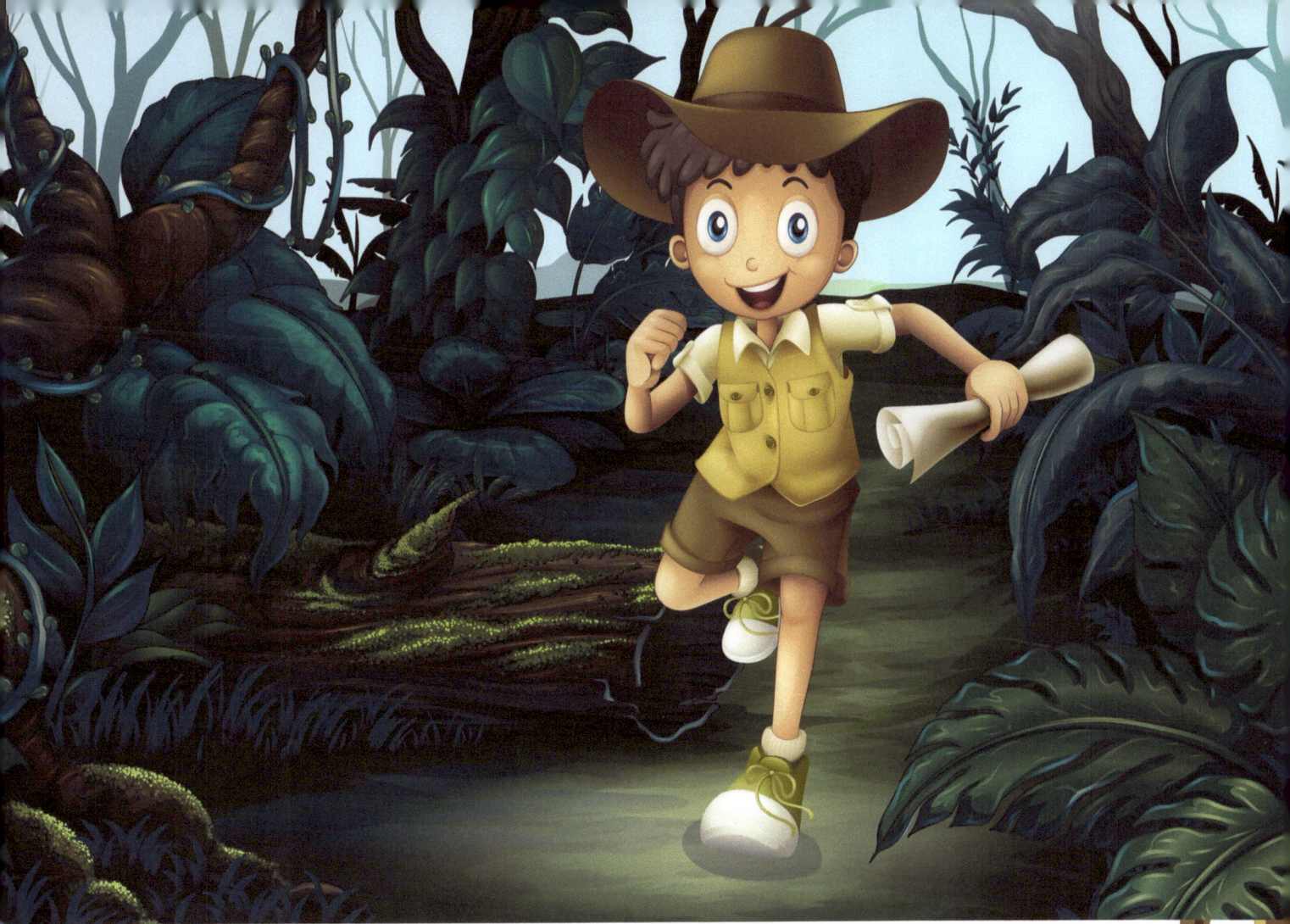

THE BOY AND THE HUNTER

Once, there lived a little boy with his mother in a small village.

One day, his mother was putting the clothes to dry in the back of their house while the boy was playing there. Since the boy was little, his mother always watched over him when he played.

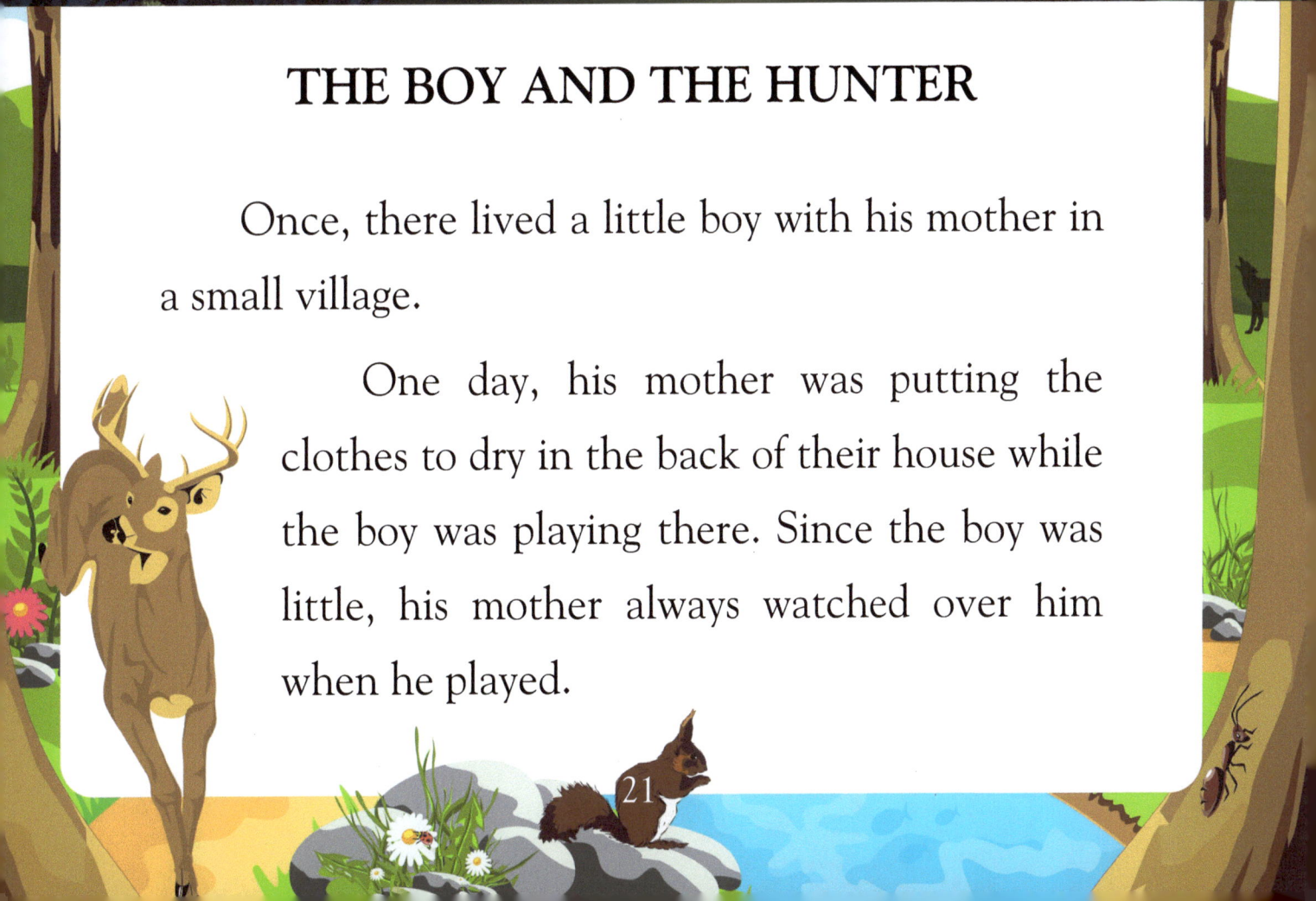

His mother told him, "I am going inside the house, and I will be back in a little while. Don't go anywhere."

The boy said, "Okay, mum."

The boy continued to play after his mother went inside the house. Then, he saw a hunter go past his house. He thought, 'Let me go behind the hunter and find out where he is going.'

And so, the boy followed the hunter. He walked behind the hunter for a long distance, and finally, they both reached the forest.

The boy began to admire the tall green trees, the lovely flowers and the birds chirping in tree tops. Hence, he did not see where the hunter was going.

The hunter had gone in another direction while the boy went in a different direction.

Now the boy was lost in the forest...

And suddenly, there appeared a lion…

The boy became scared and started to cry out loud…

The hunter heard the boy crying, so he hurried in that direction. When the hunter saw that the lion was near the boy, he shot in the air…

The lion got scared and ran away.

The hunter took the boy back to his home safely.

The boy's mother told the boy, "When I came out of the house, I noticed that you were missing. I was very worried and upset."

The boy promised his mother that from then onwards, he will always listen to her advice.

> **Moral: Always listen to your parents and elders.**

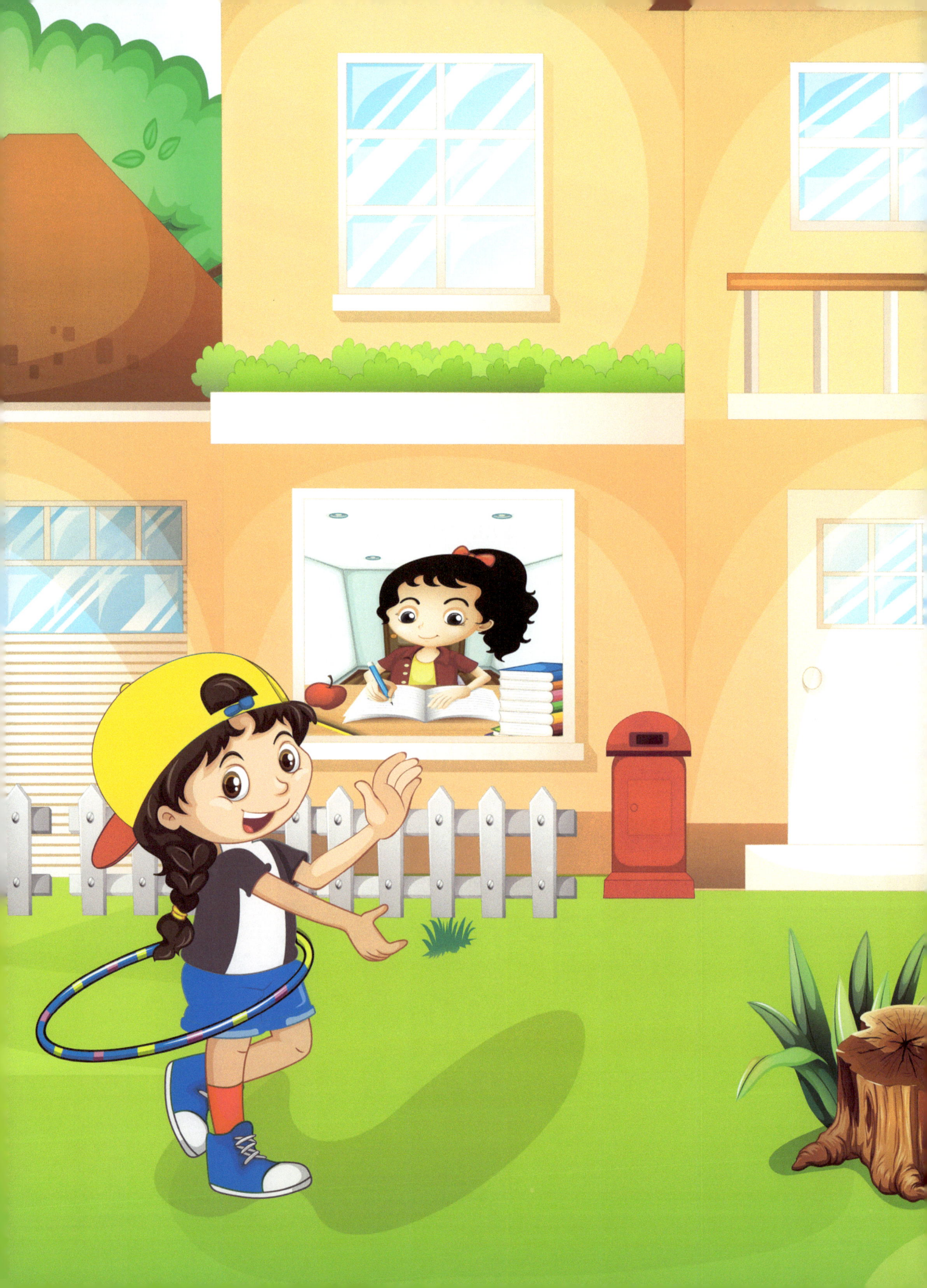

CLEVER TINA

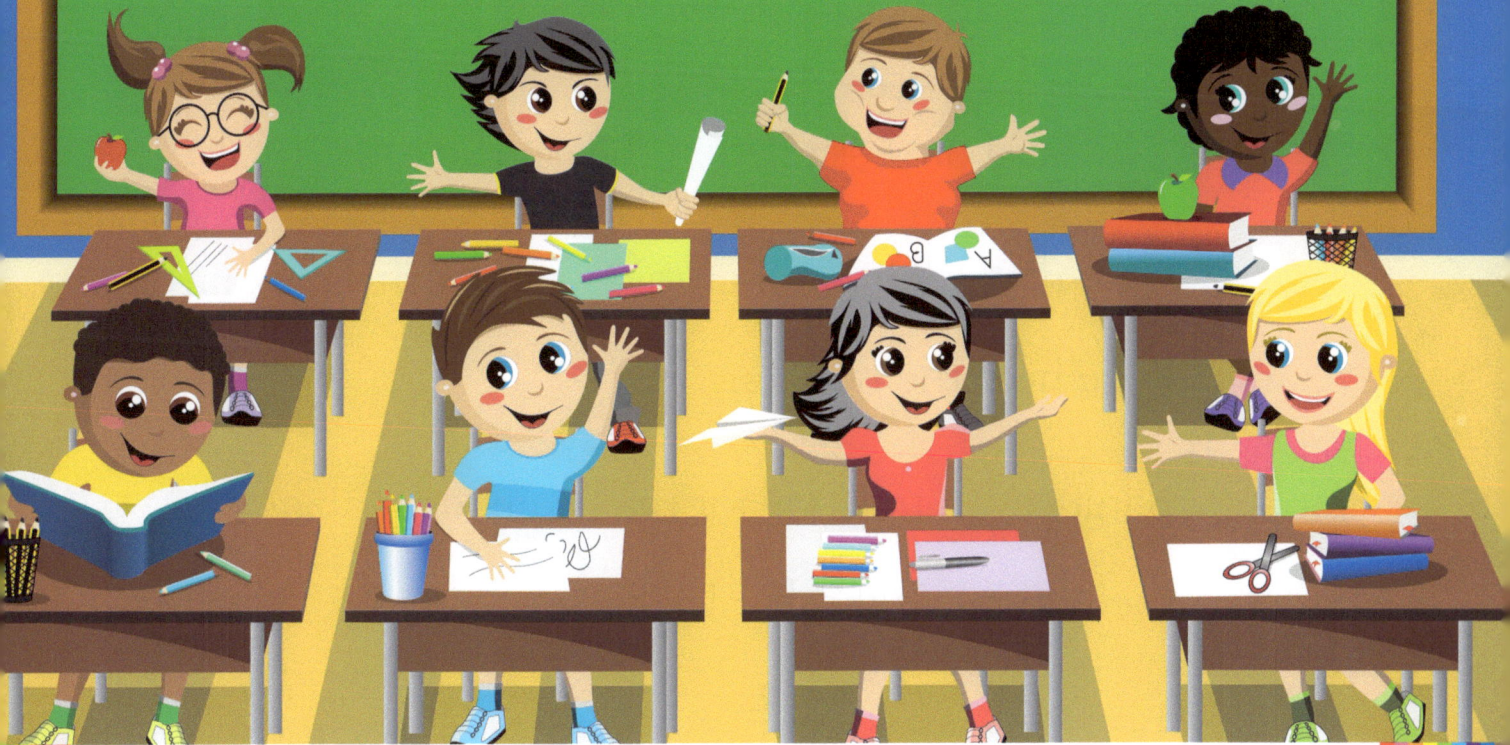

Once upon a time, there was a cute and lovable girl named Tina. She was very nice. She obeyed her elders, had good manners, and was clever and brave and also hardworking.

She was loved by all; her mother, father, brother, sister, cousins, grandparents, aunts, uncles, friends, teachers and everyone living in the village.

Her best friend's name was Sina. Sina was also very clever and hardworking and was loved by all.

Tina and Sina studied in the same class.

One day, their teacher said that a written exam would be held the next day.

Tina began to study for the exam, as soon as she returned home after school.

But Sina was not in a mood to study for the exam.

Sina thought, 'I could copy all of Tina's answers because I know that Tina would know all the answers.'

Sina went to Tina's house that afternoon.

Tina asked her, "Why did you come to play today? Did you forget that tomorrow is our exam?"

Sina said, "No, I did not forget, and I know that tomorrow is our exam."

Since Tina was smart, she thought, 'May be, Sina is thinking of copying my answers at the exam.'

Sina asked her, "Tina, what are you thinking? Come on, let's go out and play."

Tina answered, "No, you go and play, I do not want to play."

So, Sina played and enjoyed till evening. Then, when she was feeling sleepy, she went home and slept.

Tina was still awake. She stayed awake the whole night studying for the school exam.

It dawned to the next day – the day of the exam...

Sina was very happy thinking she could copy Tina's answers.

But, Tina had thought of an idea, not to let Sina copy her answers. When they reached school, Tina asked her teacher whether she could sit outside of the classroom and write for the exam.

The teacher was surprised. She asked, "Why do you want to sit outside and write for the exam?"

Tina said, "I want to sit outside because I do not want anyone to copy my answers during the exam."

The teacher agreed, and Tina sat outside the classroom.

When Sina saw this, she went to the teacher and asked, "Can I sit with Tina?"

The teacher replied, "No. Tina will sit outside for the exam. You can sit with her after the exam is over."

Sina was very scared because she had not studied for the exam.

When all the children got their exam papers, Sina read all the questions, but she did not know the answer to even one of them. She was just gazing at the questions aimlessly.

Her teacher, looked at her and asked, "What happened, Sina? Why are you not writing?"

Sina said, "Actually, I did not study yesterday. But it's okay because I know the answers to all of the questions."

The teacher understood why Sina wanted to sit with Tina and also understood Tina's plan.

In the meanwhile, Tina thought, 'Hmm... Sina will not feel good if she gets fewer marks, I think I will also get fewer marks this time, and I am sure Sina would learn a good lesson then.'

After the exam was over, the teacher collected the exam sheets of the children.

The next day, the teacher was checking all the exam papers of the students. She was astonished when she saw that what Tina had written were all wrong and had got a big 0, instead of very good marks. After that she saw Sina's exam paper - she also had got very bad marks and a big 0 on top of the paper.

The teacher started to think, and then understood that Sina got a big 0 because she had not studied for the exam. The teacher also understood Tina's plan to get bad marks in her exam paper so that Sina would learn a lesson.

When Sina found out that Tina had got a big 0, she understood that Tina had done that on purpose to teach her a lesson.

Since then, Sina always studied before her exams,

Both Tina and Sina score well in all their exams now.

Moral: Never cheat. Not even in the exams.

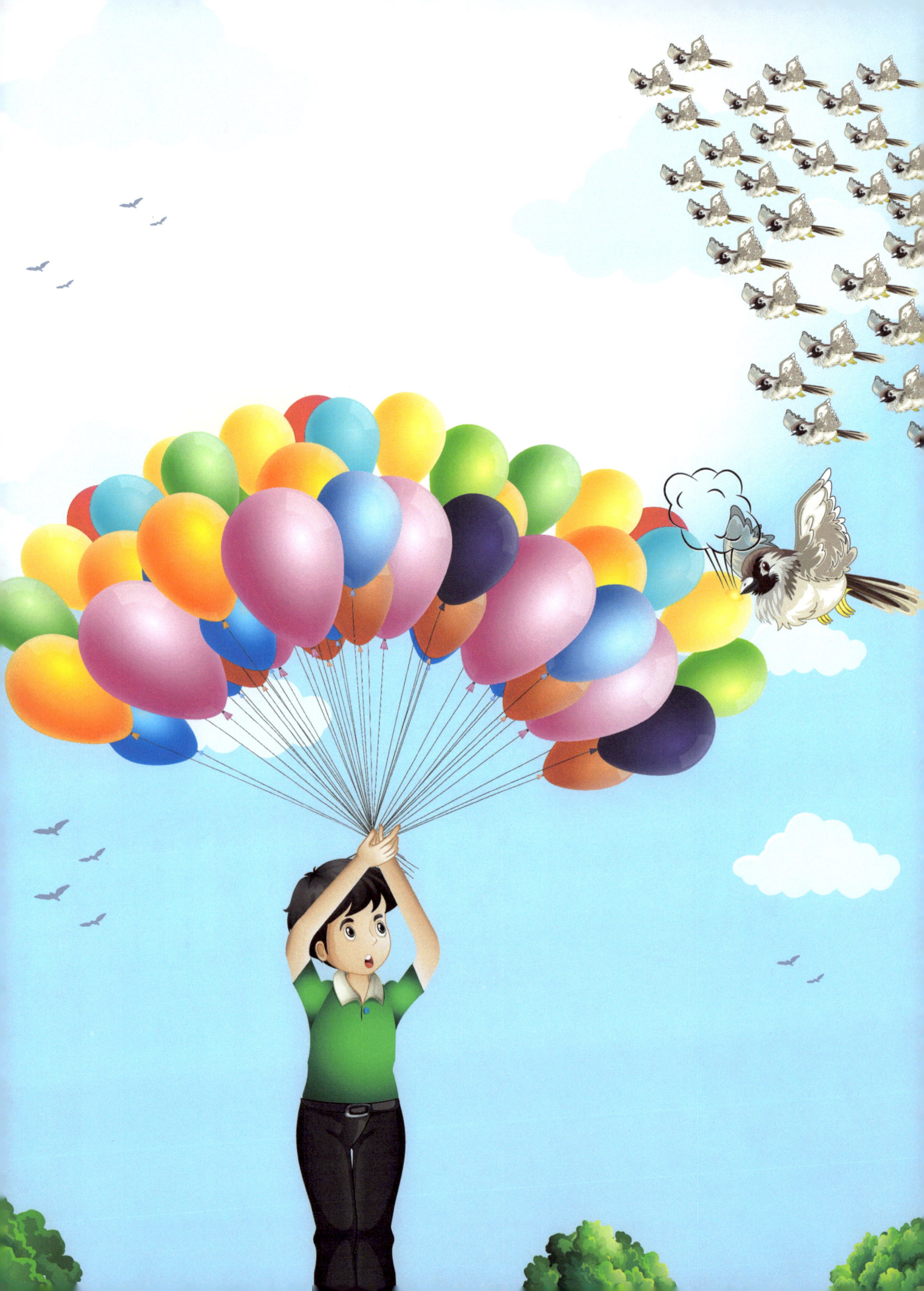

BOONU THE BALLOON SELLER – PART 1

Boonu, the balloon seller, was selling his balloons like every other day. But today he had many more balloons than ever before.

Suddenly, Boonu was carried up high into the sky by all his helium balloons!

Boonu was now floating in the sky. He was very worried that he will not be able to get back to the ground. He shouted for help, but there was no one up there to help him.

A sparrow that was flying nearby heard his cries and understood that the balloons would have to be burst so that Boonu can reach the ground.

So, with its beak, the sparrow began to burst many of Boonu's balloons.

The balloon seller thought, 'This good bird will burst all the balloons and I will go down.'

But the sparrow burst only a few balloons because after bursting a few of them she became very tired. So, the bird flew away.

The balloon seller was very sad because the bird flew away. He began to sob.

The sparrow saw that the balloon seller was very sad. She hurriedly called out to all her friends.

They all flew towards the balloon seller. Boonu was very happy.

The birds burst all of the balloons, and Boonu came down and reached the ground safely.

He thanked all of the birds for their help. He gave the birds some food. The birds ate the food and flew away.

Boonu was very happy.

Moral: Always help the ones who need your help.

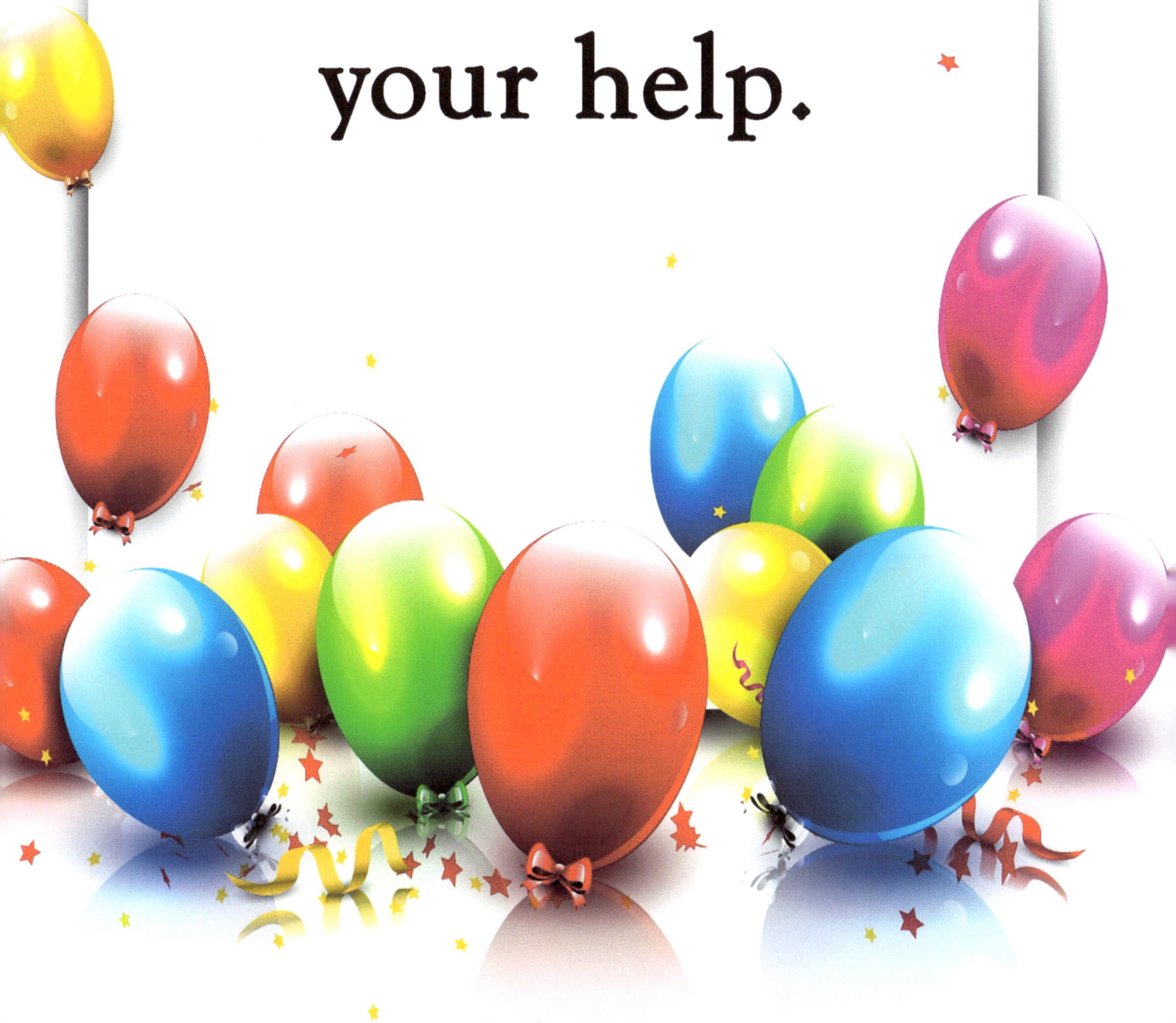

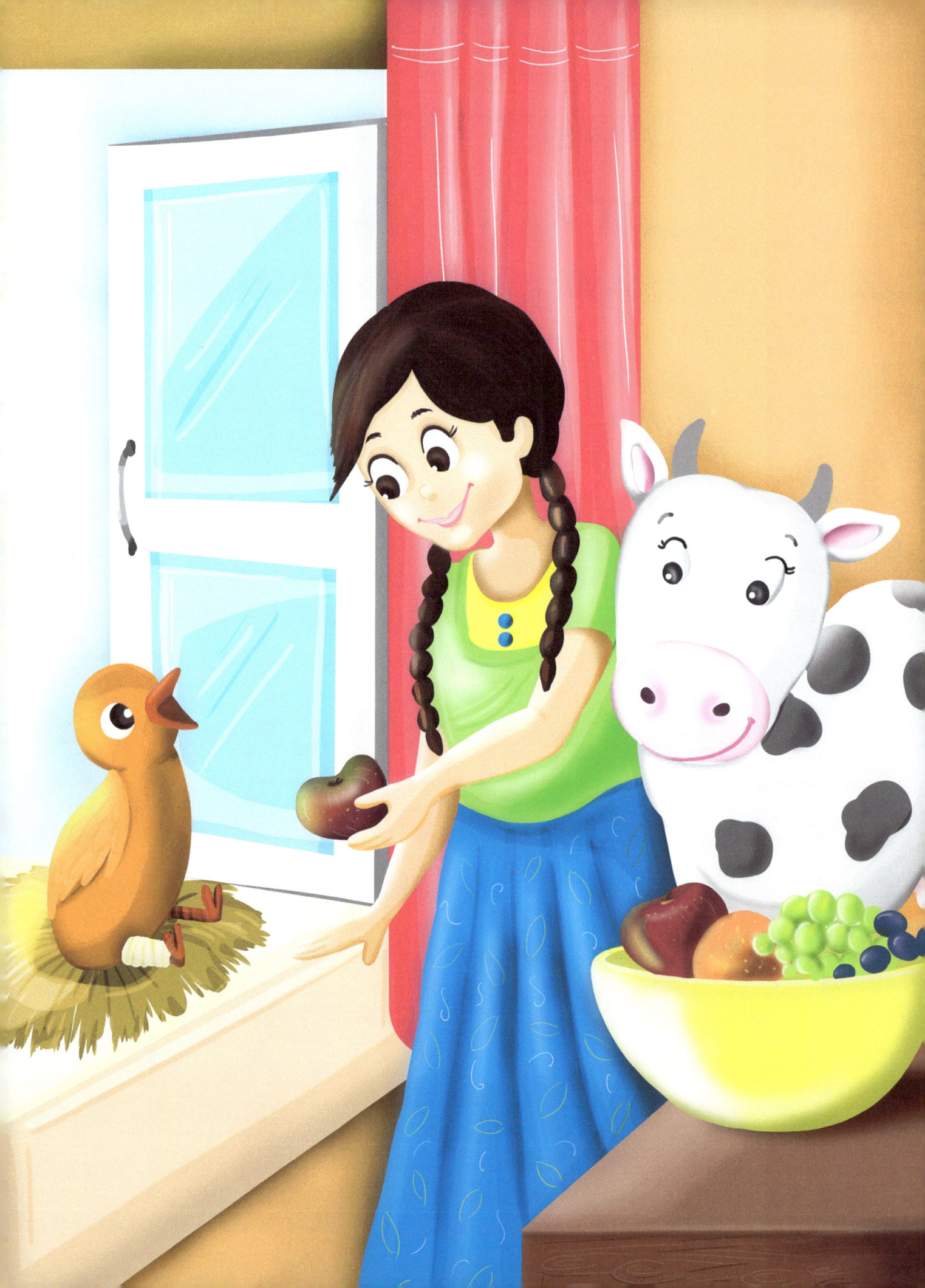

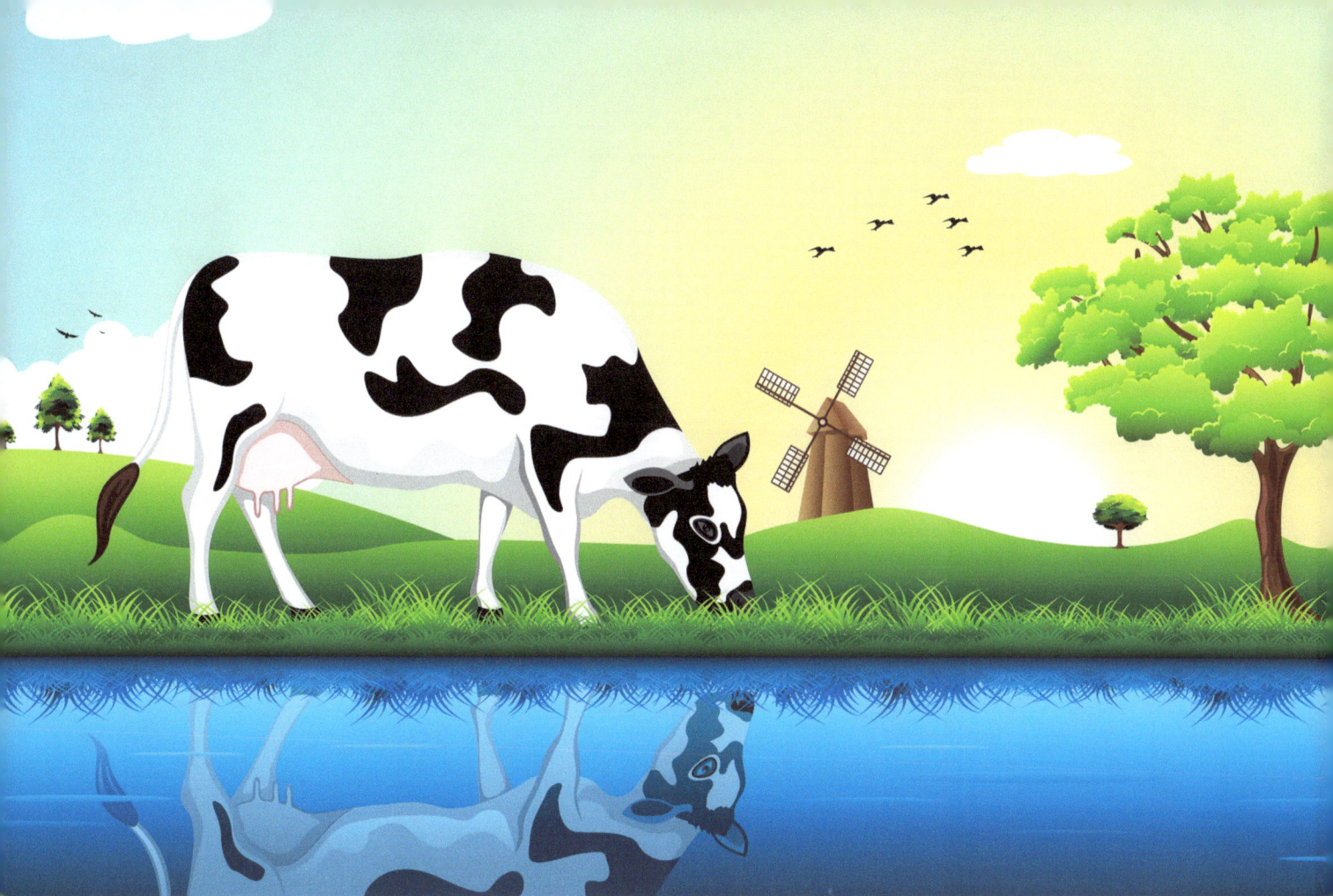

RADHA AND MITTU

Once there was a kind-hearted little girl named Radha. She had a very lovable cow named Mittu.

Radha and Mittu were best friends. Every evening, they wandered through the hills and played on the hill slopes together.

One evening, Radha said to Mittu, "Let's play wall catcher. I will run, and you catch me."

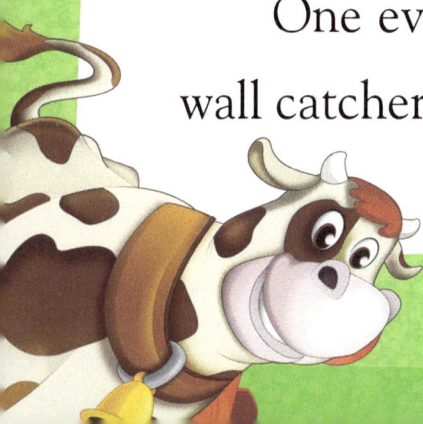

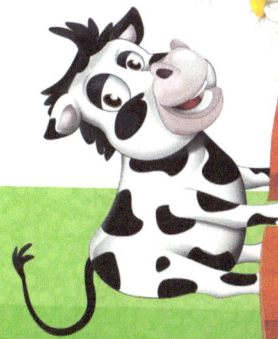

"Okay," said Mittu.

And so, they began to play. Radha ran, and Mittu chased her. They were having lots of fun playing wall catcher.

Then, suddenly, Radha saw a bird falling off from a tree top. She called out to Mittu, "Come here Mittu!"

Mittu came near her.

Radha said, "Look, there is a bird that has fallen from a tree. His leg is injured. Let's take him to our home and keep him with us until his leg gets better."

"Yes, that would be very good," said Mittu.

They took the bird to their home. They placed a bandage around the bird's injured leg, and they cared for him. They gave the bird delicious fruits to eat. They played with the bird too.

Soon, the bird was fine. The bird thanked Radha and Mittu for being so kind to him.

He flew away to his home where his friends were waiting for him. He happily played with his friends.

The bird often thought about Radha and Mittu, and he missed them. Radha and Mittu too missed the bird.

But they were all very happy.

Moral: Be kind and helpful to everyone just like Radha and Mittu.

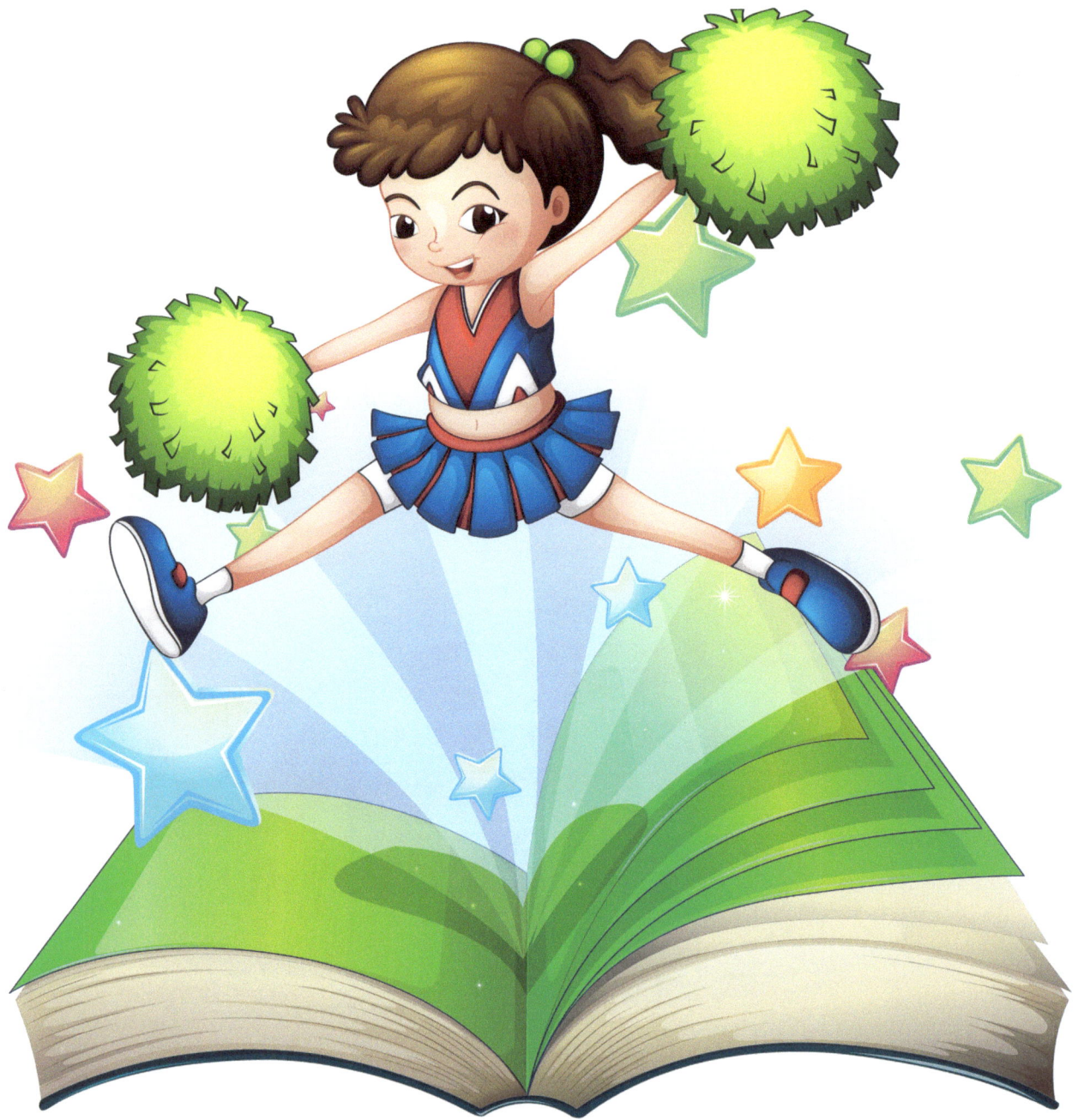

www.ingramcontent.com/pod-product-compliance
Lightning Source LLC
Chambersburg PA
CBHW052043190326
41520CB00002BA/173